SOMATIC EXERCISES
FOR BEGINNERS

Grace Vinson

COPYRIGHT

In no way is it legal to reproduce, duplicate, or transmit any part of this document electronically or in printed format. The recording of this publication is strictly prohibited. Any storage of this document is not allowed unless with written permission from the publisher.

The information provided herein is stated to be truthful and consistent. In terms of inattention or otherwise, any liability, by any use or abuse of any policies, processes, or directions contained within is the solitary and utter responsibility of the recipient reader. Under no circumstances will any reparation, damages, or monetary loss due to the information herein, either directly or indirectly

Disclaimer Notice: Please note the information contained within this document is for educational and entertainment purposes only. Every attempt has been made to provide accurate, up-to-date, reliable, complete information. However, no warranties of any kind are expressed or implied.

The reader acknowledges that the author does not render legal, financial, medical, or professional advice.

The content of this book has been derived from various sources.
Please consult a licensed professional before attempting any techniques outlined in this book.

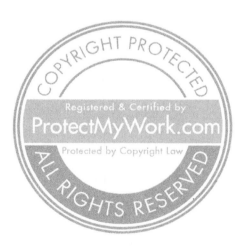

Table of contents

What is Somatic Therapy

Welcome to this journey towards well-being through somatic therapy. In a world where daily stress and tensions seem inevitable, somatic therapy stands as an accessible refuge for anyone, offering an innovative approach to improve mental and physical health. Somatic therapy embraces the fundamental idea that the mind and body are intricately connected, forming a continuum where emotional experiences are reflected in the body itself. Unlike many other therapies, the focus is not solely on the mind or body separately but on understanding their interconnection. It's a path that values awareness of bodily sensations, paving the way for a profound reconnection with oneself.

The 3 Key Pillars:

- **Mind-Body Integration:** Somatic therapy places at its core the notion that the mind and body are interdependent. Recognizing and honoring this connection is the first step towards well-being.
- **Awareness of Physical Sensations:** Through attention to bodily sensations, somatic therapy guides us to greater awareness of how emotions manifest physically.
- **Release of Stress and Tension:** Fluid movements and somatic practices aim to release stress and tension, promoting a rebalance of both body and mind.

Managing Chronic Stress through Somatic Therapy

Somatic therapy provides a comprehensive method for managing chronic stress by focusing on physical manifestations such as muscle tension, breathing patterns, and posture. This approach teaches individuals to engage actively with these responses, enhancing their ability to identify and address stress early on. Techniques such as deep breathing, guided movements, and mindful meditation are key components of this therapy. They aid in calming the nervous system and shifting the body from a state of high alert to one of relaxation and balance, which helps alleviate stress symptoms and builds resilience over time.

By equipping individuals with practical, body-focused strategies, somatic therapy not only improves daily coping mechanisms but also empowers people with a greater sense of control over their reactions to stressors. This leads to more effective and sustainable stress management.

Exploring the Connection Between Trauma and Body

The link between trauma and the body is often overlooked, yet it plays a significant role in human experience. Whether psychological, emotional, or physical, trauma leaves lasting marks on both our minds and bodies.

This section explores how our bodies retain traumatic memories and how this impacts our recovery.

Trauma overwhelms our coping mechanisms, disrupting both our physiological and psychological processes, leading to states of hyperarousal or shutdown. These reactions, rooted in our evolutionary fight-or-flight or freeze response, aim to protect us but can become maladaptive when triggered frequently or for extended periods.

Understanding how trauma is stored in the body involves grasping the concept of 'body memory,' where memories of traumatic events are retained not only in our conscious minds but also as physical sensations and patterns. While these memories may not always be accessible to our conscious awareness, they manifest physically as tension, somatic issues, and persistent pain. To alleviate these symptoms, focused movements and relaxation techniques can be employed.

Trauma often affects muscle tissue and fascia, causing tension, stiffness, and reduced flexibility.

The endocrine system, which regulates hormones, is also impacted by trauma, altering stress chemicals like adrenaline and cortisol and affecting mood, immunity, and metabolism. Additionally, trauma can affect certain brain regions involved in memory, executive function, and emotion regulation, leading to emotional instability and cognitive challenges.

Physical symptoms of trauma, known as somatic manifestations, have strong emotional and psychological components. They may trigger emotional reactions, perpetuating the trauma cycle. Addressing these bodily aspects of trauma is essential for effective treatment and healing.

Somatic exercises, including body awareness, breathing, and mindful movement practices, offer a holistic approach to releasing accumulated trauma from the body, complementing traditional talk therapies. By acknowledging and addressing these somatic components, we can enhance trauma recovery efforts, paving the way for more comprehensive healing

Overcoming Challenges in
Somatic Exercises

Embarking on Somatic Exercises can be a rewarding journey, yet it comes with its share of challenges. This chapter delves into common hurdles encountered during somatic exercises and offers practical solutions for a more fulfilling experience.

- Maintaining focus during exercises presents a significant challenge. Our minds are accustomed to constant stimulation, making it difficult to maintain the deep awareness required for Somatic Exercises.

- Creating a distraction-free environment is essential to address this issue. Practicing in a comfortable space, free from interruptions, enhances concentration. Additionally, starting each session with a few minutes of deep breathing or meditation helps center the mind for the exercises ahead.

- Managing physical sensations during exercises is another common obstacle. While some discomfort is expected, pain signals the need to pause and reassess. Beginning with gentle exercises and gradually increasing intensity allows the body to adapt safely. Listening to the body and respecting its limits is crucial for a safe and effective practice.

- Somatic exercises can evoke intense emotions, especially for those dealing with trauma or chronic stress. It's natural for feelings such as fear or anger to arise.
  Allowing these emotions without judgment is important, recognizing them as a natural part of the healing process. If emotions become overwhelming, it's advisable to pause and return to grounding techniques like deep breathing.

- Feeling frustrated with progress is another challenge. Improvement in somatic exercises takes time and consistency. Maintaining realistic expectations and celebrating small victories can help sustain motivation. Recognizing progress, no matter how small, fosters dedication to the practice.

- Some individuals may struggle with vulnerability when confronting deeply ingrained tensions and emotions. Working with a qualified somatic therapist can provide guidance and support. Therapists create a safe space for exploring vulnerabilities and integrating experiences into the healing process.
- Medical conditions or physical restrictions may present challenges. Consulting a healthcare provider before starting somatic exercises is crucial. Modifications can accommodate physical limitations while ensuring the practice remains beneficial and safe.
- Maintaining a regular practice can be challenging due to life's demands. Establishing a routine by dedicating a set time each day to somatic exercises helps build consistency.

Short sessions are better than none, and as benefits become evident, motivation to continue grows.

In conclusion, while difficulties in somatic exercises are inevitable, they are manageable. By understanding and addressing these challenges, practitioners can optimize their practice and enhance their experience. Approach these exercises with compassion, patience, and a willingness to grow. Now, let's explore the symptoms and issues that somatic therapy can help with:

- **Physical Discomfort** (Fatigue, Aches, Muscle Tension)
- **Digestive Issues** (Bloating, Gas, Diarrhea)
- **Cognitive Challenges** (Forgetfulness, Confusion)
- **Emotional Strain** (Anxiety, Depression, Irritability)
- **Sleep Disturbances** (Insomnia, Nightmares)
- **Heart and Cardiovascular Symptoms** (Chest Pain, Rapid Heartbeat)
- **Immune System Affected** (Frequent Infections)
- **Behavioral Changes** (Social Withdrawal, Communication Issues)
- **Unexplained Changes in Habits** (Weight Fluctuations, Substance Use)

If you encounter even just one of these problems, commit yourself to do your best and proceed optimistically in this new experience.

Benefits of Somatic Therapy:

Let's explore the numerous benefits resulting from consistent practice of somatic therapy:

- **Stress Reduction:** Regular practice significantly diminishes anxiety and worries, contributing to emotional equilibrium.
- **Pain Relief:** Targeted movements facilitate the release of muscular tension, alleviating chronic pain and enhancing overall quality of life.
- **Improved Sleep:** The bodily and mental relaxation promoted by somatic therapy can enhance sleep quality and support restorative nights.
- **Metabolism Boost (Indirect Benefit for Weight Loss):** While somatic therapy isn't a direct weight loss program, its impact on stress can indirectly improve metabolism. Reducing stress may facilitate weight loss, as lower cortisol levels contribute to a more efficient metabolism.
- **Increased Flexibility and Mobility:** Fluid movements promoted by somatic therapy improve flexibility and joint mobility.
- **Enhanced Emotional Balance:** The bodily awareness developed through this practice contributes to greater emotional stability and improved psychological well-being.

Discover Well-being, Wherever You Are

Designed to be accessible to all, our somatic exercises extend an invitation to discover well-being. Perform them outdoors for a purely immersive experience, or recreate a tranquil environment at home to fully enjoy the convenience of this therapy. Indeed, all you need is a mat and a bit of space, and wherever you are, you can immerse yourself in this extraordinary journey of self-discovery.

Somatic exercises find their primary space on the floor. Whether in a reclined or seated position, the floor plays a pivotal role in these exercises by providing valuable insights into our body. It acts as a medium for perceiving how our body moves, a skill referred to as proprioception.

Our emphasis lies in experiencing the sensations within our body, prioritizing the feeling over its appearance.

In the upcoming section, we will begin exploring each somatic exercise.
Taking them one at a time, we'll delve into the movements and sensations, ensuring unwavering focus to attain a sense of well-being. Following that, we will incorporate these exercises into a dedicated month-long somatic therapy program

Before we begin, **please turn to page 71, the third-to-last page of the book, where you'll find the QR code.**

By scanning it, you'll gain access to a comprehensive collection of videos where each somatic exercise is broken down step by step and performed by one of my students.
This resource will guide you through the exercises, ensuring proper execution and maximizing the benefits of the program.

Plus, you'll unlock a second bonus, which we'll discuss later.

I really would like to hear your thoughts about your experience because your input is valuable and can inspire those who want to start this rewarding journey.

If you have a moment, please consider leaving a review.

FLOOR STAR

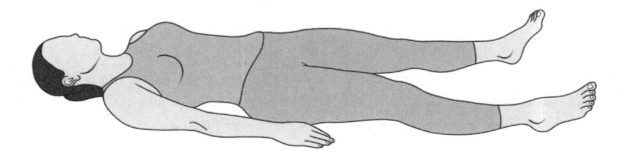

The Floor Star exercise is critically important as it forms the cornerstone of your entire workout regimen. It emphasizes the crucial role of controlled breathing and maintaining a conscious, mindful connection with every part of your body. Regularly engaging in this exercise helps you establish a solid foundation for a comprehensive and effective fitness routine.

Integrating this exercise into your daily morning routine can be tremendously beneficial. By dedicating just two minutes each morning to this practice, you can significantly enhance your day with a boost of positivity and energy.

If you're feeling particularly stressed or tense, extending the duration of this exercise can help amplify its soothing effects, helping to calm your mind and body more profoundly.

How to Perform It:

- Begin by lying down on your back on a comfortable surface, such as a yoga mat or a softly carpeted area. Make sure that your legs are spread slightly wider than shoulder-width apart, and lay your arms down along your sides in a relaxed posture.
- Take a moment to really center yourself, focusing deeply on your breathing. Aim to completely relax your body and ensure you are fully present in the moment. Inhale slowly through your nose, then exhale gently through your mouth, feeling your body sink deeper into relaxation with each breath.
- Pay close attention to every point where your body contacts the floor. Feel the support of the ground beneath your head, shoulders, back, hips, and legs. Identify any spots where you feel tension or discomfort.
- Observe the natural curve of your spine. Adjust your feet to find a comfortable position, ensuring that your legs remain loose and unstrained. Make any necessary adjustments to maximize your comfort and ensure proper body alignment.
- Continue to breathe deeply and intentionally. With every inhale, imagine your body filling with calm and rejuvenating energy. As you exhale, picture all your tension and stress evaporating.
- Maintain this pattern of focused breathing until you establish a strong, harmonious connection between your body and the floor. This sense of alignment prepares you to transition smoothly to subsequent exercises.

Benefits:

- Increases awareness of each body part, enhancing your ability to monitor your physical state from head to toe.
- Grounds you in the present moment, which is essential for cultivating mindfulness and reducing everyday stress.
- Acts as an effective preparatory exercise, setting the stage for more dynamic or demanding activities in your routine.

BABY STRETCH

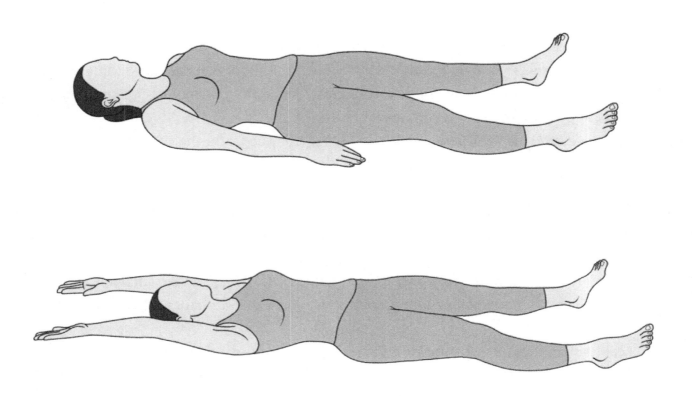

The Baby Stretch is a wonderfully effective exercise, specially designed to elongate the body and alleviate tension that accumulates due to stress and past traumas. Such conditions often lead to muscle stiffness, making this exercise an ideal choice for those looking to release pent-up negative emotions and rejuvenate their energy levels.

Mimicking the natural stretching of an infant, this exercise emphasizes the innate simplicity and effectiveness of the movements involved. If the movements feel challenging, it could indicate a particular need for the kind of emotional and physical release this exercise provides.

How to Perform It:

- Begin by lying flat on your back, ensuring your legs are spread wider than shoulder-width and your arms are extended straight beside you.
- Take a deep breath and slowly raise your arms overhead while simultaneously stretching your legs out, imagining the gentle, awakening stretch of a baby.
- Hold this extended pose for about 5 seconds, maintaining a rhythm in your breathing to enhance the stretch's effectiveness.
- Carefully and slowly return to your starting position, ensuring your movements remain controlled and smooth throughout the exercise.

Benefits:

- Enhances Physical Flexibility: Regularly performing the Baby Stretch can significantly improve your flexibility, making daily activities feel easier and more fluid.
- Boosts Emotional Well-Being: By releasing tension and fostering relaxation, this exercise contributes positively to your emotional health, helping you feel more balanced and less stressed.
- Improves Posture and Body Alignment: The Baby Stretch also aids in aligning and correcting your posture, contributing to better overall body mechanics and reducing the likelihood of pain and injury in daily life.

This exercise is simple yet powerful, offering profound benefits not just physically, but emotionally as well, making it a valuable addition to any daily routine.

PELVIC PREPARATION

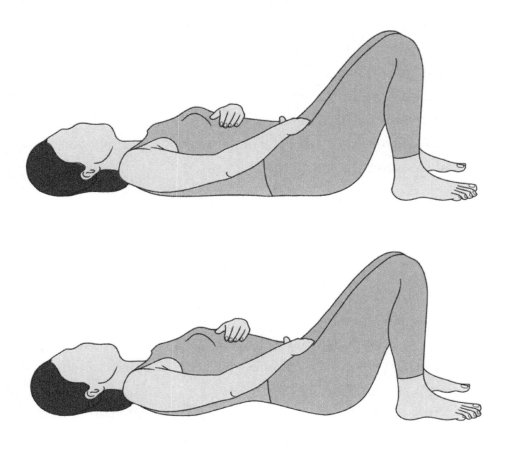

The Pelvic Preparation exercise is a therapeutic movement designed to enhance the connection with your pelvis and lower back, shifting your focus towards a deeper understanding of breath control and body awareness.

This exercise encourages you to inhale deeply while arching the back and to exhale while relaxing, facilitating the release of worries and tensions. This process not only aids in physical relaxation but also promotes emotional calm. The unique method of breathing and moving that Pelvic Preparation introduces serves to enrich your overall well-being and body harmony.

How to Perform It:

- Begin by sitting on the ground with your knees bent and feet firmly planted.
- Place one hand just above your navel, extending towards the ribs, and position the other hand below the navel, touching the top of the pelvis, to better feel the movements of your core.
- Imagine your tailbone as a paintbrush, with the ground beneath you acting as a canvas. This visualization helps you conceptualize the movement of your lower back as an artistic expression, where each motion paints a stroke on the imaginary canvas.
- As you inhale, initiate a 'painting' motion with your tailbone, gently arching your lower back as if drawing an upward curve on the canvas behind you.
- As you exhale, gently round your spine forward, as if pulling the brush towards you, which helps elongate and relax the back into the ground, completing the curve on your canvas.
- Continue this breathing pattern, synchronizing your breath with the movements: arching the spine on the inhale and rounding it on the exhale, maintaining a smooth and rhythmic flow throughout the exercise.

Benefits:

- Enhances spine flexibility and body awareness: The rhythmic movements involved in this exercise increase spinal flexibility and heighten bodily sensations and control.
- Promotes profound relaxation: By focusing on deep, controlled breathing and deliberate movements, this exercise fosters significant relaxation and stress relief.
- Improves overall spine mobility: Regular practice of the Pelvic Preparation exercise helps to loosen and strengthen the spine, aiding in better mobility and pain reduction.
- Builds a stable foundation: This exercise strengthens the pelvic region, establishing a stable foundation that supports overall balance and posture.

The Pelvic Preparation exercise is an excellent way to connect deeply with your body's core, engaging both mind and muscles in a practice that not only alleviates physical tension but also enhances mental clarity and focus.

EAGLE POSE

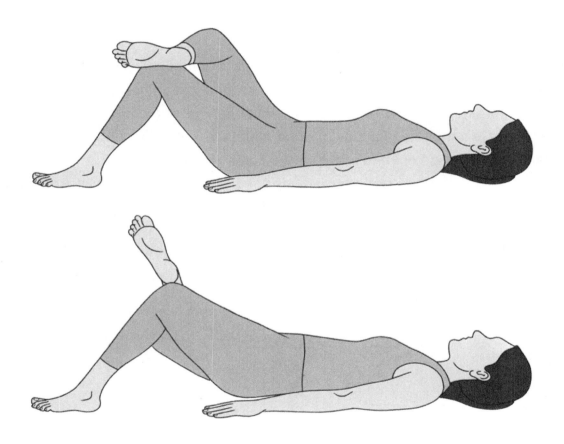

The "Eagle Pose" is a dynamic and complex exercise specifically designed to improve mobility in the lower body and enhance flexibility in the back. This pose actively encourages muscle relaxation, especially effective during exhalation, helping to release accumulated physical and mental tension.

Although it may initially appear challenging, the benefits and techniques of the Eagle Pose become clear once demonstrated, ideally viewed through our video course accessible by scanning the QR code on page 71.

How to Perform It:

- Start by lying on your back with your arms at your sides and palms facing down, bending your legs with feet firmly planted on the ground.
- Bend your right leg and place the outside part of your right ankle on your left knee, creating a slight stretch in the right glute.
- Keep your arms slightly open on the floor to aid in maintaining balance throughout the exercise.
- Keep your back firmly on the ground as you rotate your hips to the right, guiding your right ankle towards the floor while simultaneously bringing your relaxed left leg towards the right side.
- Proceed at a comfortable pace, focusing intently on your breathing; inhale as you return to the starting position, and exhale deeply as you perform the rotation.
- Complete the sequence by repeating the movement on the opposite side, swapping the positions of your legs to ensure balance in muscle engagement and flexibility enhancement.

Benefits:

- Increases mobility in the lower body and back.
- Encourages relaxation of all muscles, with a special emphasis on exhaling to release tension.
- Aids in dissipating stress and promoting a sense of ease.

The Eagle Pose not only aids in physical conditioning but also serves as a therapeutic tool to unwind and release stress, making it a valuable component of any fitness regimen focused on holistic well-being.

MOVING ROCK

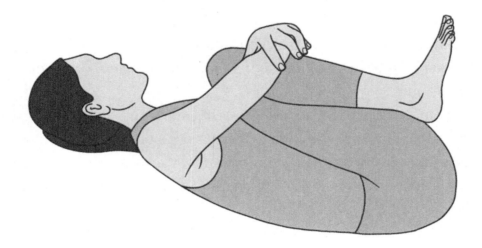

The Moving Rock exercise is skillfully designed to enhance both balance and flexibility, specifically targeting the abdominal muscles for core strengthening. This movement not only helps in releasing tension but is also effective in preventing and alleviating lower back pain.

As you perform this exercise, focus on the sensation of release and allow yourself to let go of stress and stiffness, embracing the soothing motion.

How to Perform It:

- Begin by lying on your back and gently bring your knees towards your chest, following any visual guidance provided.
- Gently rock your body from side to side, maintaining balance throughout the movement. This rocking should feel pleasant and effortless, ensuring your spine remains in constant contact with the mat.
- Continue alternating the movement from one side to the other, moving slowly to maximize the effectiveness of the exercise and enhance the engagement of your core muscles.

Benefits:

- Improves balance and flexibility, helping you achieve greater physical coordination and ease of movement.
- Engages the abdominal muscles, which is essential for building core strength and stability.
- Facilitates the release of tension in the lower back, contributing significantly to both the prevention and relief of back pain.

The Moving Rock exercise is an excellent way to integrate gentle yet effective movements into your routine, promoting a healthier spine and a more flexible body while also providing a calming and stress-relieving experience.

NECK AND HIPS

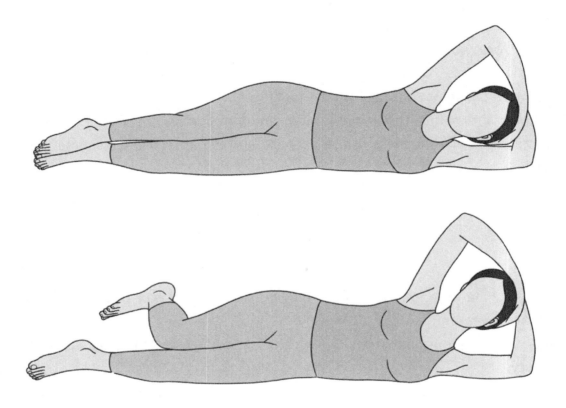

The Neck and Hips exercise is specifically designed to strengthen and enhance flexibility in the neck and hip areas. As you engage in this sequence, lying on your side, it's crucial to pay close attention to the nuances of each movement and position, fostering a mindful connection with your body.

This exercise not only focuses on physical conditioning but also emphasizes the synchronization of movements, which is essential for overall coordination and muscle engagement.

How to Perform It:

- Start by lying in a fetal position on your left side, bending your knees to approximately 90 degrees. Use your right hand as support between your right cheek and the mat, ensuring stability and comfort.
- Extend your left hand over your head, and as you do so, elevate your head using your left hand to create a stretch along the right side of your neck. Concurrently, lift your left ankle while maintaining alignment with your knees to enhance the stretch in your hip area.
- Hold this stretched position for about 2 seconds, allowing your muscles to fully engage and stretch.
- Gently revert to the starting fetal position and prepare to repeat the exercise on the opposite side, ensuring even conditioning and flexibility on both sides of your body.
- Throughout the exercise, maintain a focus on fluid transitions between positions and synchronize the movements of your neck and hips. Keep your breathing steady and deep to enhance the mind-body connection and maximize the benefits of the exercise.

Benefits:

- Strengthens the neck, hips, and glutes, while simultaneously improving their flexibility. This dual focus helps in preventing injuries and enhancing movement efficiency.
- Enhances overall coordination and engages often overlooked muscles, which is vital for maintaining balance and functional strength in everyday activities.
- Contributes to hip stability and provides relief from neck, low back, and hip discomfort, offering a comprehensive approach to alleviating common pain points.

The Neck and Hips exercise is an excellent way to address key areas that are crucial for mobility and pain relief, making it a valuable addition to any fitness regimen focused on holistic health and flexibility.

CHEST OPENING

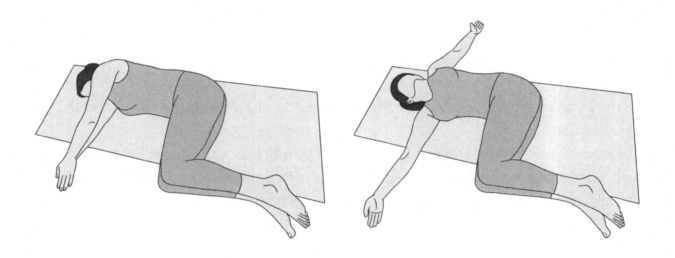

The Chest Opening exercise is a targeted routine designed to enhance the flexibility of your chest and shoulders while promoting better coordination. This exercise places a special emphasis on mindful breathing, which significantly enhances the rejuvenation and opening of the upper body.

The movement involved in the Chest Opening not only facilitates physical expansion but also serves as a therapeutic release for accumulated tension.

How to Perform It:

- Begin in a fetal position on your right side, extending your right arm forward on the ground for support, and placing your left hand above it.
- Envision your left hand tracing a semicircle in the air. Initiate the chest opening by sweeping the left hand through the air, keeping your right hand grounded. As you start this motion, inhale deeply to prepare your body for the stretch.
- Continue the sweeping motion until your left hand touches the floor on the opposite side, effectively creating a wide opening across your chest. Hold this position for a moment and take a deep breath in to maximize the stretch.
- As you exhale, slowly return to the starting position, feeling the stretch and relief build in your upper body with each repetition. This controlled breathing helps integrate the physical movement with relaxation and release of tension.
- Finish the routine by performing the same fluid movement on the opposite side, ensuring to inhale as you open and exhale as you return to start. This helps to maintain balance and a thorough engagement of the muscles involved.

Benefits:

- Enhances the flexibility of the chest and shoulders, allowing for a greater range of motion and easing movements that may have been restricted.
- Provides an effective method for releasing tension in the upper body, which is crucial for alleviating stress and promoting relaxation.
- Contributes to improved posture and overall body alignment by strengthening and loosening the chest area, which often becomes tight from daily activities like sitting or computer work.

The Chest Opening exercise is an excellent way to open up the body's core areas, promote healthful breathing, and enhance physical posture and flexibility, making it a valuable component of any wellness or fitness routine.

DESPAIR

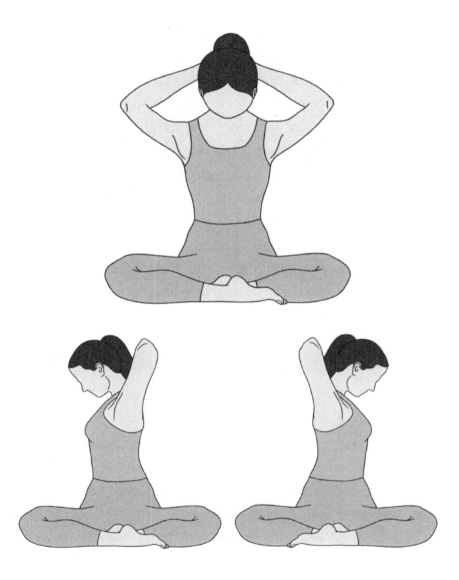

The Despair exercise is designed to address feelings of distress and discouragement by focusing on the neck and upper body, areas often harboring emotional tension. This exercise aims to provide emotional release and stress reduction. Importantly, it can be adapted for those who find sitting on the floor uncomfortable; it can be equally effective when performed while seated in a chair.

How to Perform It:

- Begin by sitting on the mat with your legs crossed, or if preferable, sit on a chair to ensure comfort. Keep your back upright to promote proper posture throughout the exercise.
- Place both hands gently on the back of your head. Slowly lower your head forward until your chin touches your collarbone, finding a position that feels comfortable and sustainable, whether on the mat or in the chair.
- As you maintain your hands on the back of your head, slowly turn your face to the left, inhaling deeply to stretch the sides of your neck and the upper body.
- Exhale gently as you return to the initial forward-facing position. Repeat the sequence on the opposite side to complete a full cycle of the exercise. Ensure each movement is smooth and synchronized with your breathing to maximize the release of tension.

Benefits:

- Effectively addresses feelings of distress and discouragement, offering a physical method to cope with emotional upheavals.
- Enhances flexibility in the neck and upper body, areas critical for maintaining good posture and reducing physical tension.
- Accommodates various comfort levels, as it can be performed just as effectively on a chair, making it accessible to a wider range of individuals.
- Targets emotionally tense areas, significantly contributing to overall stress reduction and emotional well-being.

The Despair exercise not only helps in alleviating emotional stress but also improves physical flexibility and comfort, making it a valuable practice for those dealing with emotional and physical strains.

ROLL IN

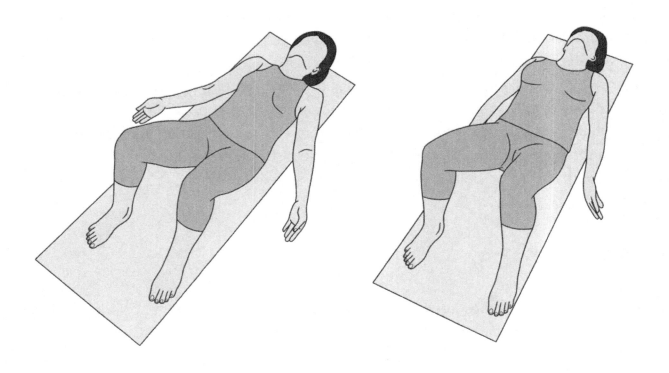

The "Roll In" exercise is designed to significantly enhance shoulder flexibility and mobility. This exercise is pivotal for those looking to improve their upper body range of motion and ease movements that involve the shoulders.

By integrating the Roll In into your routine, you can expect to see gradual improvements in how your shoulders move and feel, especially if you spend a lot of time at a desk or performing tasks that don't involve extensive shoulder movement.

How to Perform It:

- Begin by lying on your back with your legs bent and feet flat on the ground. Position your arms slightly wider than your hips to ensure a stable base for the movement.
- Start the exercise by inhaling gently and turning your palms to face inward, preparing your body for the movement.
- As you exhale, smoothly roll your arms outward, ensuring your palms and forearms stay in contact with the ground. Simultaneously, gently tilt your chin upwards towards the ceiling, aligning your neck with the spinal movement to enhance the stretch.
- Continue to perform this movement slowly and with control, focusing on the sensation of your shoulders rotating and the stretch it provides. The coordination of breath with movement is crucial for maximizing the effectiveness of this exercise.

Benefits:

- Improves shoulder flexibility and mobility, aiding in better ease of movement and less restriction during daily activities or other upper body exercises.
- Enhances upper body coordination, helping synchronize movements and improve overall body control.
- Relieves stress and tension in the shoulders and upper back, promoting a more relaxed posture and reduced discomfort.

This exercise is especially beneficial for those looking to enhance their upper body's responsiveness and ease discomfort related to stiffness or limited mobility in the shoulders.

Consistent practice will help you grasp the dynamics of the movement and experience the associated benefits more profoundly.

ROLL OUT

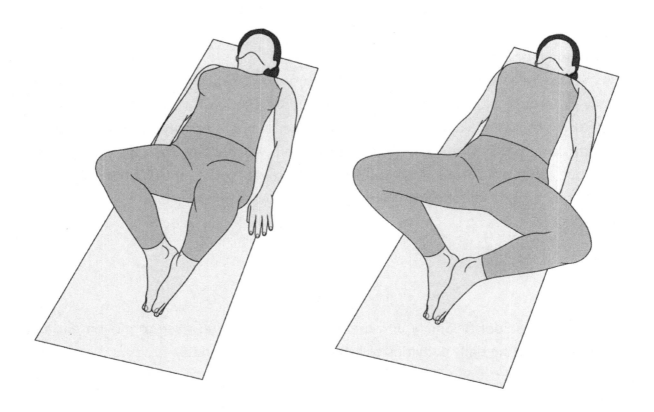

The "Roll Out" exercise focuses on enhancing the flexibility and mobility of the groin and lower back areas. This movement is crucial for anyone looking to increase their range of motion and alleviate tension in these critical regions.

Let's explore the steps to effectively perform this beneficial exercise, which combines controlled movements with focused breathing for optimal results.

How to Perform It:

- Start by lying on your back with your legs bent and feet flat on the ground. This will be your starting position.
- Exhale deeply as you gently let your knees drop outward, bringing the soles of your feet to face each other. This motion should be slow and controlled to avoid any strain.
- Hold this position for two seconds, allowing your muscles to adjust to the stretch. If you find the stretch too intense, adjust your legs outward to a more comfortable position where the tension is minimal yet effective, and hold for two seconds.
- Inhale as you slowly bring your knees back up to the starting position, focusing on the movement and your breath to maximize the benefit of the exercise.

Benefits:

- Regularly performing the Roll Out exercise significantly improves flexibility and mobility in the groins and lower back, areas that are crucial for overall bodily movement.
- By focusing on controlled breathing and avoiding unnecessary muscle contraction, this exercise helps to execute movements smoothly, which is essential for maintaining a healthy back.
- The Roll Out not only alleviates tension but also contributes to better posture by strengthening the muscles around the spine and lower body.
- This exercise encourages a deeper connection with your body, helping you become more attuned to your physical needs and limitations.

Incorporating the Roll Out into your routine offers multiple health benefits, promoting greater bodily awareness and flexibility while helping to maintain a pain-free lower back.

SPINAL WAVE

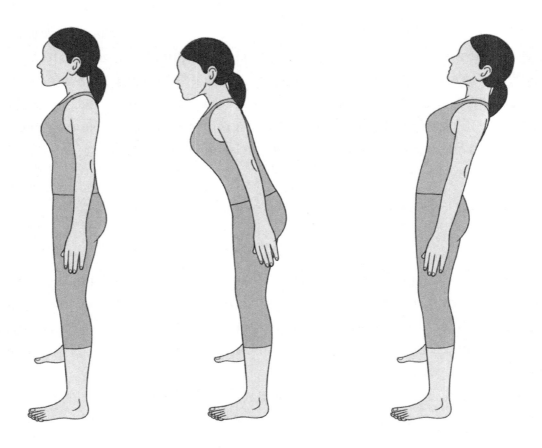

The "Spinal Wave" exercise is designed to significantly enhance the mobility and flexibility of the spine. This exercise is crucial for anyone looking to improve their spinal health and ensure smooth, pain-free movements throughout the day. By practicing the Spinal Wave, you will engage in a fluid, wave-like motion that not only helps to prevent stiffness but also strengthens the mind-body connection.

How to Perform It:

- Start in a standing position with your arms relaxed at your sides, ensuring your body forms a straight line.
- Begin the exercise by gently moving your upper chest forward, then return it to the starting position. As you do this, simultaneously move your pelvis and belly forward to continue the wave-like motion through your body.
- Focus on the fluidity of the movement, allowing each segment of your spine to follow in a smooth, wave-like pattern. This continuity is key to fully engaging the spinal muscles and joints.

Benefits:

- Greatly improves spine mobility and flexibility, which can help reduce the risk of pain and stiffness in the back area.
- Helps release tension within the spinal muscles, enhancing the overall smoothness and ease of movement. Consistent practice leads to better posture and fewer muscle imbalances.
- Recognized as one of the most effective exercises for promoting back health and strengthening the mind-body connection, the Spinal Wave encourages a deeper awareness of your spinal alignment and movement patterns.

Incorporating the Spinal Wave into your exercise routine can provide profound benefits for your spinal health, enhancing both your physical flexibility and mental focus.

REACH BACK

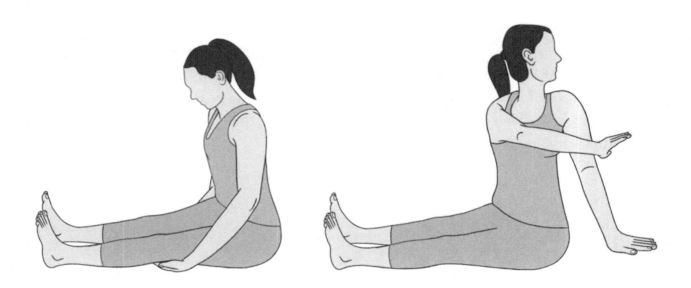

The "Reach Back" exercise is strategically designed to enhance the mobility and flexibility of the upper back, shoulders, and lower back.

This position targets crucial areas that are often neglected, providing a comprehensive workout that improves overall upper body function and stress relief.

How to Perform It:

- Begin by sitting on the mat with your legs extended straight in front of you. Ensure that your posture is upright and your spine is aligned.
- Keeping your legs stationary, twist your upper body to the left. This movement should be smooth and controlled, focusing on the rotation from your upper spine.
- Place your left hand on the mat for support and reach backward with your right hand, extending through your shoulders and upper back.
- Return gently to the starting position and then repeat the movement on the opposite side, alternating sides to ensure balanced development of flexibility and strength in the upper body.
- Throughout the exercise, maintain a focus on relaxation and controlled breathing. Deep inhales and exhales will optimize the stress-release benefits and help maintain a calm, focused mind during each stretch.

Benefits:

- Increases mobility and flexibility in the upper back, shoulders, and lower back, which is vital for overall spinal health and ease of movement.
- Encourages the body to remain relaxed and the legs to stay stationary while executing the twisting motion, which enhances the effectiveness of the stretch and prevents unnecessary strain.
- Utilizes one arm on the mat for balance, which ensures stability during the exercise and helps in maintaining proper form.
- Deep exhales during the stretch help in the complete release of tension and trauma, enhancing stress relief and promoting a more relaxed state post-exercise.

This exercise is excellent for those looking to improve their spinal health, relieve stress, and enhance the flexibility of their back and shoulders. The Reach Back not only benefits physical health but also contributes to mental well-being by encouraging mindfulness and breath control.

STANDING REACH

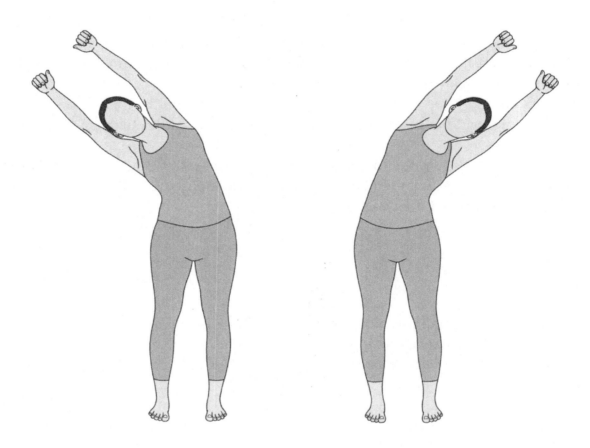

The "Standing Reach" exercise is designed to enhance the flexibility and mobility of the upper body, while also fostering a heightened sense of connection and balance.

This exercise is ideal for improving overall upper body strength and flexibility, and for enhancing coordination and spatial awareness.

How to Perform It:

- Begin by standing upright with your feet shoulder-width apart and your hands resting by your sides.
- Slowly extend your arms overhead and lean towards the left side, ensuring that your feet remain firmly planted on the ground and your legs stay straight.
- Gradually move your hands and torso in front of you, creating a smooth semi-circle motion with your arms.
- Continue this slow and controlled movement until you reach the right side. Then, reverse the motion in the opposite direction to complete one full repetition.
- Focus on executing each movement with deliberate and intentional actions. Maintain controlled breathing and ensure your body stays relaxed throughout the exercise. It's important to avoid rushing through the movements to maximize their benefits. Pay special attention to keeping your neck relaxed and not tensed up during the exercise.

Benefits:

- Increases flexibility and mobility in the upper body.
- Enhances the sense of connection and balance with your body.
- Controlled breathing throughout the exercise contributes to a mindful and effective practice.

This exercise actively engages the muscles of the upper body while promoting relaxation and mindfulness, making it a beneficial addition to any fitness routine. Regular practice can lead to significant improvements in both physical and mental well-being.

SPIDER CIRCLE

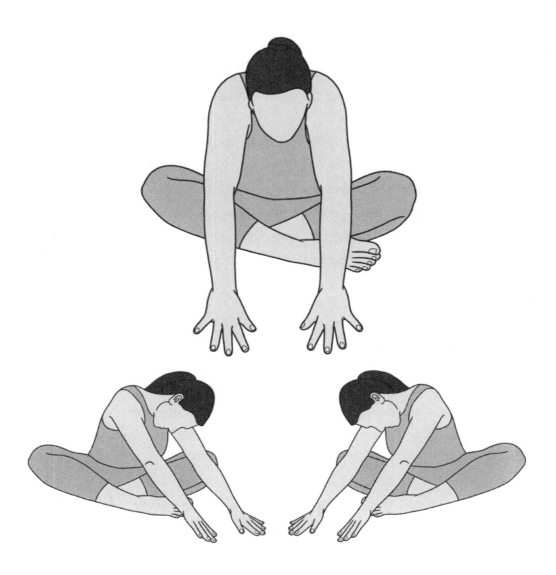

The "Spider Circle" exercise is uniquely designed to enhance upper body flexibility, alleviate tension, and provide emotional relief. This exercise differs from traditional stretches like the "Standing Reach" by incorporating a circular motion that promotes a unique release of negative energy and tension.

Engaging in this rhythmic exercise allows you to experience a deep sense of surrender, helping you let go of accumulated stress effectively.

How to Perform It:

- Begin by sitting on a mat in a crossed-legged position, leaning forward slightly to start the motion.
- Reach your hands toward the floor directly in front of you, initiating the movement with your upper body.
- Execute a smooth and controlled 90-degree clockwise rotation, extending your hands as far as possible while maintaining balance and alignment in your spine.
- Complete the circle by continuing the rotation until you return to your starting position.
- After completing the rotation clockwise, repeat the circular movement in a counterclockwise direction to ensure balanced muscular engagement and flexibility enhancement.

Benefits:

- Improves upper body flexibility, especially in the neck, which is crucial for reducing stiffness and enhancing mobility.
- Increases flexibility in the glutes and lower back, contributing to overall spinal health and posture improvement.
- Emphasizes the relaxation of the neck; it's important to keep the neck relaxed and avoid tensing it during the exercise to maximize the benefits.
- Focuses on emotional release, offering significant relief from traumas and accumulated tension, which can often manifest physically in the body.
- Facilitates the release of negative energy and encourages a sensation of surrendering, which can be profoundly calming and rejuvenating.

This exercise is an excellent way to address physical stiffness and emotional stress simultaneously, making it a beneficial addition to any holistic wellness routine. Regular practice can lead to improved flexibility, reduced tension, and enhanced emotional well-being.

STAR GLUTE BRIDGE

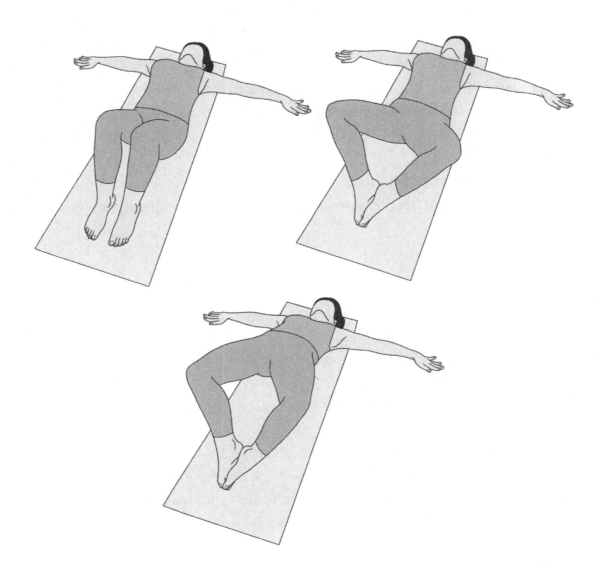

The "Star Glute Bridge" exercise is an excellent routine designed to strengthen the glutes and groins while also promoting a gentle stretch in the groin area.

This exercise combines rhythmic movement with deep breathing, offering both physical and relaxation benefits. Ideal for enhancing lower body stability, the Star Glute Bridge also helps in tension release through controlled breathing.

How to Perform It:

- Begin by lying on your back with your knees bent and feet together on the floor, forming a 90-degree angle with your arms extended along your sides.
- Inhale deeply and allow your knees to drop sideways, bringing the soles of your feet together. Feel the gentle opening in your groin area and hold this position for 3 seconds, maintaining stability and focus on your core.
- Inhale again and engage your glutes to lift your hips upwards, keeping your soles together and knees open, while your arms remain extended to maintain balance.
- Exhale fully as you slowly lower your buttocks back to the mat, controlling the movement to return your knees to the starting bent position.
- Focus on performing slow, controlled motions and maintaining continuous breathing throughout the exercise to maximize effectiveness and relaxation.

Benefits:

- Strengthens the glutes and groins, which are essential for overall lower body stability and support.
- Encourages deep breathing, which aids in tension release and promotes relaxation during the exercise.
- Maintains core engagement throughout the exercise, helping to stabilize and strengthen the core muscles.
- Provides a gentle stretch in the groin area, enhancing flexibility and reducing the risk of injury in this sensitive region.

This exercise is beneficial for those looking to improve lower body strength, enhance core stability, and release tension effectively through mindful movement and breathing.

STANDING STRESS RELEASE

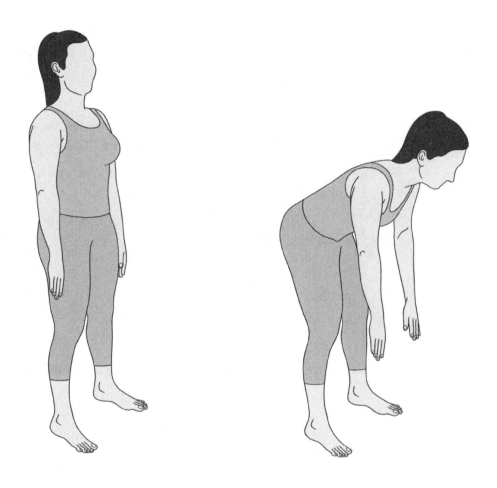

The "Standing Stress Release" exercise is a simple yet profoundly effective technique designed to alleviate tension and foster relaxation. By focusing on gentle shaking and twisting of the upper body, this exercise allows you to release negative emotions and stress.

It's a perfect routine for those seeking both mental and physical liberation through movement.

How to Perform It:

- Start by standing on a mat with your feet slightly wider than shoulder-width apart to ensure stability.
- Allow your upper body to relax completely. Let your arms hang loosely, and let your head and shoulders gently collapse forward, maintaining engagement in your lower body to keep your balance.
- Hold this relaxed, collapsed position for 5 seconds, letting any tension in your neck, shoulders, and arms melt away.
- Slowly return to your initial standing position, feeling rejuvenated and lighter as you rise.

Benefits:

- Facilitates the release of tension and stress, helping to unwind the knots that build up in the upper body.
- Encourages a profound sense of mental and physical relaxation, making it easier to let go of the day's stresses.
- Focuses on the importance of mental clarity and emptying the mind, enhancing your ability to release worries during the exercise.
- Enhances the flexibility of the upper body through gentle, controlled twisting and turning, promoting better movement and flexibility.
- Promotes a holistic approach to stress relief by addressing both physical tension and mental burdens.

This exercise is ideal for those moments when you need a quick but effective way to shed stress and rejuvenate both your mind and body. Regular practice can significantly enhance your overall well-being and ability to handle stress.

FULL BODY ROCKING

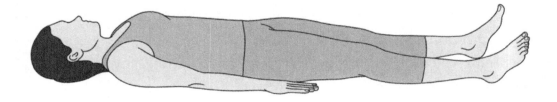

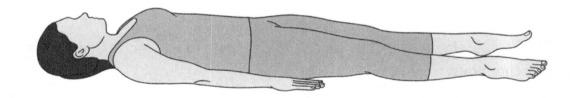

The "Full Body Rocking" exercise is a holistic and dynamic sequence that encourages you to engage every part of your body in a rhythmic and coordinated manner.

This exercise is not just a physical activity but a profound experience that harmonizes the rhythm of your breath with the motion of your body, creating a seamless dance from your toes to your head. It invites you to delve into the artistry of movement, enhancing your connectivity with yourself.

How to Perform It:

- Start by lying on your back on a comfortable surface, with your legs spread slightly wider than shoulder-width apart and your arms resting by your sides.
- Begin the sequence by inhaling slowly and lifting your toes while holding the breath for 5 seconds. This initial action sets the tempo for the rhythmic movement to follow.
- Transition into exhaling slowly, extending your toes away from you, as if pushing a gentle wave of energy through your body, for 3 seconds.
- Continue this fluid sequence, synchronizing your breath with the movement of your toes. Let each cycle be smooth and controlled, creating a dance-like rhythm that flows through your entire body.

Benefits:

- Cultivates a rhythmic connection throughout the entire body, enhancing physical coordination and mental focus.
- Infuses each breath with softness and revitalizing energy, rejuvenating your body with every cycle.
- Nurtures an innate awareness of the body's entirety, fostering a natural synchronization between movement and breath.
- Elevates the integration of breath and movement, offering a uniquely holistic experience that benefits both mind and body.
- Guides you on a mindful journey from your toes to the crown of your head, forging profound mind-body unity and enhancing overall wellbeing.

The Full Body Rocking exercise is a beautiful way to integrate mindful breathing with dynamic physical movement, making it an excellent practice for those looking to deepen their connection to their body and enhance their overall sense of well-being.

STRETCH AND COMPRESS

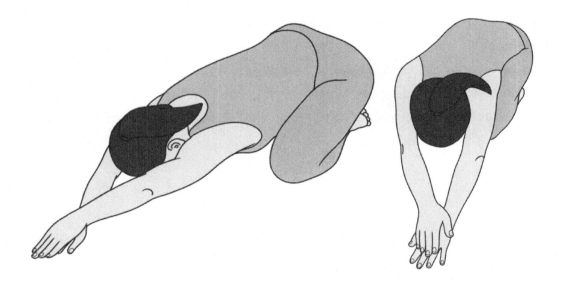

The "Stretch and Compress" exercise is specifically designed to enhance mobility and alleviate tension in the back. Drawing inspiration from primitive and natural postures, this exercise is particularly beneficial for individuals who spend long periods sitting, as it effectively counters the stiffness and discomfort associated with such lifestyles.

How to Perform It:

- Start by sitting back on your shins with your heels directly beneath your hips, ensuring your spine is upright to foster proper posture.
- Extend your arms forward on the ground in front of you to begin the stretch.
- Shift slightly to the left, reaching your left arm further to the side while placing your right hand gently on your left wrist to deepen the stretch.
- Hold this position for 10 seconds, focusing on the stretch along your back and the side of your body.
- Gently return to your starting position and then repeat the stretch on the right side by extending your right arm and using your left hand to enhance the stretch.
- Continue to alternate between sides, maintaining a smooth and controlled movement throughout the exercise.

Benefits:

- Improves overall mobility, helping to enhance your range of motion and flexibility.
- Promotes relaxation in the back, effectively reducing tension and the potential for discomfort.
- Supports knee and ankle health by engaging and strengthening the muscles around these joints, which can often become weakened from prolonged periods of sitting.
- Offers a therapeutic exercise that is ideal for individuals accustomed to sitting for extended periods, helping to reverse the negative effects of such a sedentary lifestyle.
- Facilitates a sense of surrender and connection with your body, encouraging mindfulness and bodily awareness.

The Stretch and Compress exercise is a simple yet powerful way to reconnect with your body, offering significant benefits for both physical and mental health. Regular practice can lead to improved flexibility, reduced tension, and a better overall sense of well-being.

ENERGY OPENING

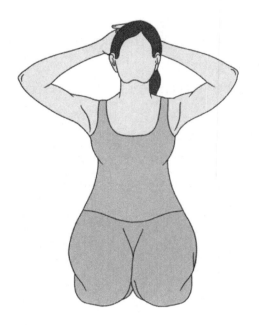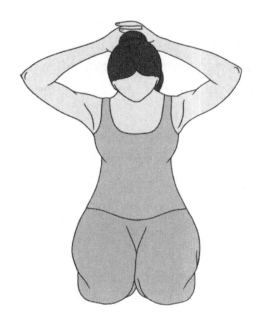

The "Energy Opening" exercise is an invigorating routine designed to enhance mental clarity and physical well-being by synchronizing controlled breathing with deliberate movements.

This exercise helps in releasing accumulated tension and fostering a deep sense of presence, making it ideal for those looking to rejuvenate their energy and focus.

How to Perform It:

- Begin by sitting on your shins with your back straight to ensure a proper posture.
- Place your hands behind your head, interlocking your fingers for support.
- As you exhale, gently lower your chin towards your collarbone, allowing the tension in your neck and upper back to release.
- Inhale deeply, lifting your head while simultaneously opening your elbows and expanding your chest to enhance the stretch.
- Hold this open, expanded position briefly to feel the flow of energizing energy, then exhale slowly as you return to your initial posture.
- Repeat this cycle, focusing on the rhythm of your breathing and the sensations of opening and releasing throughout your body.

Benefits:

- Alleviates anxiety and promotes a heightened sense of presence, helping to clear the mind and reduce stress.
- Improves neck and back health through deliberate movements that stretch and strengthen these areas.
- Supports knee health by maintaining a natural seated position, which can be beneficial for those who spend extended periods sitting.
- Encourages the release of worries and intrusive thoughts, allowing for a focus on revitalizing energy within the body, promoting a sense of renewal and clarity.

This exercise is particularly beneficial for those looking to integrate a mindful practice into their routine to enhance both mental and physical health, providing a powerful tool for stress relief and self-care.

KNEE HOLD

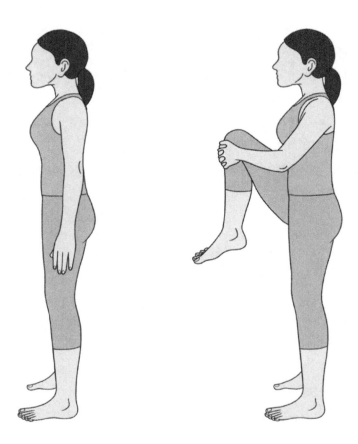

The "Knee Hold" exercise is specially designed to improve coordination, balance, and lower body mobility. By engaging in this movement, individuals can focus on their center of gravity, thus enhancing control over both body and emotions.

This exercise combines physical engagement with focused breathing to provide a stabilizing and empowering experience.

How to Perform It:

- Stand upright with your feet shoulder-width apart to ensure a stable base.
- Lift one knee towards your chest and cradle it with both hands, securing a firm but gentle grip. Keep your opposite foot firmly planted on the floor to maintain balance.
- Adopt a relaxed posture throughout your upper body, allowing your arms to fully support the weight of your lifted leg.
- Engage in deep and controlled breathing, syncing each inhale and exhale with the movement of lifting and holding your knee.
- If maintaining balance proves challenging, you can perform this exercise with your back against a wall for added support.
- Hold the knee in this position for 5 seconds, focusing on maintaining a gentle and consistent breathing rhythm.
- Gently lower your leg back to the floor and repeat the exercise with the other leg.

Benefits:

- Enhances coordination, balance, and mobility in the lower body, essential for daily activities and overall physical health.
- Promotes empowerment, allowing individuals to feel in control of their body and emotions, enhancing a sense of self-efficacy and confidence.
- Fosters a positive emotional experience through the comforting sensation of 'hugging' the knee, which can provide emotional comfort and stress relief.
- Contributes to upper body strength development while primarily focusing on the lower body, as it also engages the arms and core.

This exercise is a valuable addition to any fitness routine, offering both physical and emotional benefits that contribute to improved well-being and enhanced control over body mechanics.

NECK RELEASE

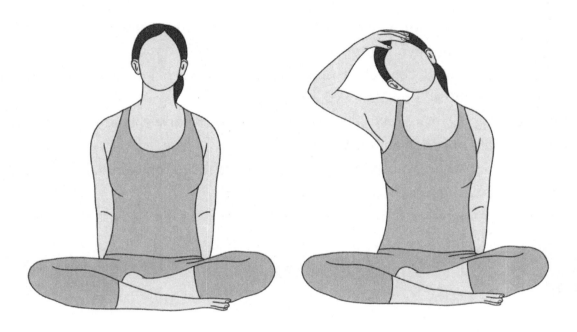

The "Neck Release" exercise is designed to promote neck flexibility and release tension through controlled and deliberate movements.

This practice not only aims to alleviate stress but also to enhance your overall sense of well-being by revitalizing the neck muscles.

How to Perform It:

- Begin by sitting on a mat with your legs crossed and your back straight and aligned, ensuring good posture.
- Extend your right hand over and place it gently on the left side of your head.
- Gently pull your head towards your right shoulder, feeling a stretch along the left side of your neck.
- Hold this position for 5 seconds, maintaining gentle and rhythmic breathing to maximize relaxation.
- Slowly release the stretch and return to the initial sitting position.
- Repeat the sequence on the opposite side by extending your left hand over your head and gently pulling the right side of your head towards your left shoulder.

Benefits:

- Releases stress and increases energy levels, contributing to a more relaxed and energized state.
- Alleviates neck tension, enhancing feelings of relaxation and reducing overall physical stress.
- Improves flexibility, posture, and alignment in the neck, which is especially beneficial for individuals who frequently engage in activities that may strain the neck, such as prolonged use of electronic devices.

Regular practice of the Neck Release exercise can significantly improve neck health and flexibility, making it a valuable addition to any daily routine focused on maintaining and enhancing physical well-being.

OPEN LIFE

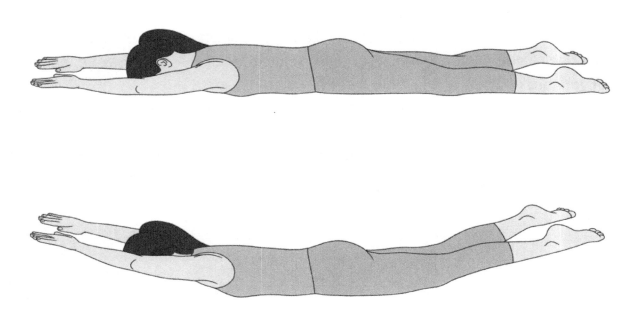

The "Open Life" exercise is a rejuvenating practice designed to align your physical and mental realms. This exercise extends beyond simple physical activity, integrating a deep symbolic meaning with the physical movements.

It begins with a posture that invites relaxation and transitions into a dynamic motion that symbolizes taking charge and building strength, enhancing both energy and happiness.

How to Perform It:

- Start by lying on your belly on a comfortable mat, with your legs extended and arms stretched forward.
- Inhale deeply and simultaneously lift your arms and legs off the mat, keeping your pelvis and core engaged with the ground. This movement should be smooth and controlled.
- Hold this lifted position for 2 seconds, feeling the strength building in both your upper and lower body.
- Exhale as you gently lower your arms and legs back to the starting position on the mat.

Benefits:

- Boosts overall energy and promotes a sense of happiness, revitalizing your mood and energy levels.
- Strengthens both the upper and lower body, enhancing muscle tone and endurance.
- Improves posture and body alignment, fostering a deeper connection with your heart and aiding in overall physical balance and stability.

Regular practice of the Open Life exercise can lead to significant improvements in your physical strength, posture, and emotional well-being, making it a holistic exercise for anyone looking to enhance their fitness and mental clarity.

28-DAY PLAN

Now that you've gained a solid understanding of each movement, it's time to embark on a transformative journey with our 28-day somatic exercise program.

This carefully curated program is designed to bring you incredible benefits with just a few minutes of commitment each day. Imagine dedicating a small portion of your time to these exercises, and in return, experiencing profound improvements in your well-being.

Over the next 28 days, these simple yet powerful exercises will become a valuable part of your daily routine. They are not just movements; they are a pathway to releasing tension, enhancing flexibility, and fostering a deep connection with your body. By investing just a few minutes each day, you are taking a proactive step towards a healthier, more vibrant you.

Let this program be your daily ritual, a time you set aside to prioritize your well-being. As you progress through the days, observe the positive changes in your physical and mental state. Whether it's increased flexibility, reduced stress, or improved overall vitality, each day brings you closer to a better version of yourself.

WEEK 1

DAY 1

Exercise	Duration/Reps
Floor Star	2 minutes
Baby stretch	6-8 reps
Chest Opening	10 reps (5 per side)
Standing Reach	10 reps
Spinal Wave	8-10 reps
Knee Hold	12 reps (6 per side)

DAY 2

Exercise	Duration/Reps
Floor Star	2 minutes
Pelvic preparation	8-10 reps
Eagle Pose	8 reps (4 per side)
Spider Circle	10 reps (5 per side)
Star Glute Bridge	8-10 reps
Standing Stress Release	12 reps

DAY 3

Exercise	Duration/Reps
Floor Star	2 minutes
Standing Reach	10 reps
Stretch and Compress	8-10 reps
Open Life	12 reps
Full Body Rocking	10 reps

DAY 4

Exercise	Duration/Reps
Floor Star	2 minutes
Roll In	12 reps
Roll Out:	12 reps
Chest Opening	10 reps (5 per side)
Moving Rock	8-10 reps

DAY 5

Exercise	Duration/Reps
Floor Star	2 minutes
Roll In	8-10 reps
Roll Out:	8 reps (4 per side)
Chest Opening	8 reps (4 per side)
Moving Rock	8-10 reps

DAY 6

Exercise	Duration/Reps
Floor Star	2 minutes
Reach Back	10 reps (5 per side
Spider Circle	10 reps (5 per side
Full Body Rocking	10 reps
Standing Stress Release	12 reps
Standing Reach	10 reps

DAY 7

Exercise	Duration/Reps
Floor Star	2 minutes
Knee Hold	12 reps (6 per side)
Star Glute Bridge	8-10 reps
Roll In	12 reps
Roll out	12 reps
Open Life	12 reps

WEEK 2

DAY 8

Exercise	Duration/Reps
Floor Star	2 minutes
Baby stretch	6-8 reps
Pelvic preparation	8-10 reps
Eagle Pose	8 reps (4 per side)
Moving Rock	8-10 reps
Spinal Wave	8-10 reps

DAY 9

Exercise	Duration/Reps
Floor Star	2 minutes
Despair	8-10 reps
Neck and hips	8 reps (4 per side)
Neck Release	8 reps (4 per side)
Stretch and Compress	8-10 reps
Energy Opening	8-10 reps

DAY 10

Exercise	Duration/Reps
Floor Star	2 minutes
Roll In	12 reps
Roll Out	12 reps
Chest Opening	10 reps (5 per side)
Moving Rock	8-10 reps

DAY 11

Exercise	Duration/Reps
Floor Star	2 minutes
Pelvic preparation	8-10 reps
Eagle Pose	8 reps (4 per side)
Star Glute Bridge	8-10 reps
Standing Stress Release	12 reps

DAY 12

Exercise	Duration/Reps
Floor Star	2 minutes
Standing Reach	10 reps
Stretch and Compress	8-10 reps
Energy Opening	8-10 reps
Full Body Rocking	10 reps

DAY 13

Exercise	Duration/Reps
Floor Star	2 minutes
Reach Back	10 reps (5 per side)
Spider Circle	10 reps (5 per side)
Knee Hold	12 reps (6 per side)
Roll Out	8-10 reps
Spinal Wave	8-10 reps

DAY 14

Exercise	Duration/Reps
Floor Star	2 minutes
Full Body Rocking	12 reps
Despair	8-10 reps
Neck and hips	8 reps (4 per side)
Neck Release	8 reps (4 per side)
Open Life	8-10 reps

WEEK 3

DAY 15	
Exercise	**Duration/Reps**
Floor Star	2 minutes
Baby stretch	8-10 reps
Chest Opening	12 reps (6 per side)
Standing Reach	12 reps
Spinal Wave	10-12 reps
Knee Hold	12 reps (6 per side)

DAY 16	
Exercise	**Duration/Reps**
Floor Star	2 minutes
Pelvic preparation	10-12 reps
Eagle Pose	10 reps (5 per side)
Spider Circle	12 reps (6 per side)
Star Glute Bridge	10-12 reps
Standing Stress Release	14 reps

DAY 17

Exercise	Duration/Reps
Floor Star	2 minutes
Standing Reach	12 reps
Stretch and Compress	10-12 reps
Open Life	14 reps
Full Body Rocking	12 reps

DAY 18

Exercise	Duration/Reps
Floor Star	2 minutes
Roll In	14 reps
Roll out	14 reps
Chest Opening	12 reps (6 per side)
Moving Rock	10-12 reps

DAY 19

Exercise	Duration/Reps
Floor Star	2 minutes
Despair	10-12 reps
Neck and hips	10 reps (5 per side)
Neck Release	10 reps (5 per side)
Energy Opening	10-12 reps

DAY 20

Exercise	Duration/Reps
Floor Star	2 minutes
Reach Back	12 reps (6 per side)
Spider Circle	12 reps (6 per side)
Full Body Rocking	12 reps
Standing Stress Release	14 reps
Standing Reach	12 reps

DAY 21

Exercise	Duration/Reps
Floor Star	2 minutes
Knee Hold	14 reps (7 per side)
Star Glute Bridge	10 reps
Roll In	14 reps
Roll Out	14 reps
Open Life	14 reps

WEEK 4

DAY 22

Exercise	Duration/Reps
Floor Star	2 minutes
Baby stretch	10 reps
Pelvic preparation	12 reps
Eagle Pose	10 reps (5 per side)
Moving Rock	12 reps
Spinal Wave	12 reps

DAY 23

Exercise	Duration/Reps
Floor Star	2 minutes
Despair	14 reps
Neck and hips	12 reps (6 per side)
Neck Release	12 reps (6 per side)
Stretch and Compress	10 reps
Energy Opening	10 reps

DAY 24

Exercise	Duration/Reps
Floor Star	2 minutes
Roll In	14 reps
Roll Out	14 reps
Chest Opening	12 reps (6 per side)
Moving Rock	10 reps

DAY 25

Exercise	Duration/Reps
Floor Star	2 minutes
Pelvic preparation	10 reps
Eagle Pose	12 reps (6 per side)
Star Glute Bridge	10 reps
Standing Stress Release	14 reps

DAY 26

Exercise	Duration/Reps
Floor Star	2 minutes
Standing Reach	12 reps
Stretch and Compress	10 reps
Energy Opening	12 reps
Full Body Rocking	10 reps

DAY 27

Exercise	Duration/Reps
Floor Star	2 minutes
Reach Back	12 reps (6 per side)
Spider Circle	10 reps (5 per side)
Knee Hold	12 reps (6 per side)
Roll Out	10 reps
Spinal Wave	10 reps

DAY 28

Exercise	Duration/Reps
Floor Star	2 minutes
Full Body Rocking	14 reps
Despair	10 reps
Neck and hips	10 reps (5 per side)
Neck Release	10 reps (5 per side)
Open Life	10 reps

After completing the 28-day somatic exercise plan, it's time to pause and reflect on how these exercises have helped us. Here are some direct testimonials from participants in the program:

- **John**: "I used to experience sudden stress and hunger attacks, which often affected my overall well-being. After incorporating somatic exercises into my daily routine, I noticed a significant decrease in stress and an improved ability to manage my emotions. Now I feel more peaceful and have started leading a healthier lifestyle, including a balanced diet and regular physical activity."
- **Sarah**: "My posture has always been a problem for me, and I often experienced back and neck pains. After following the somatic exercise plan, I noticed a significant improvement in my posture and body awareness. Now I feel more upright and free from the chronic pains that used to bother me."
- **Michael**: "I had been suffering from chronic pain for years and couldn't find relief with conventional treatments. After starting somatic exercises, I experienced significant pain relief and increased flexibility in my movements. Now I can enjoy a more active and pain-free life, thanks to this practice."
- **Emma**: "Before the program, I struggled with anxiety and had trouble sleeping. The breathing and movement exercises introduced in this plan helped me calm my mind and improved my sleep quality dramatically. I now feel more rested and less anxious."
- **Lucas**: "As someone who sits at a desk all day, I used to feel sluggish and had frequent headaches. These somatic exercises have really revitalized my energy levels and reduced my headaches significantly. I'm more productive and energetic."
- **Sophia**: "Dealing with emotional instability was challenging for me. Through this program, I've learned how to ground myself and deal with emotional upheavals more effectively. It's truly been a life-changing experience."

These testimonials demonstrate the transformative power of somatic exercises and their ability to improve the quality of life for those who regularly practice them.

Bonus Extra

In previous chapters, we've explored the significant impact of physical activity on our mind-body connection and overall well-being.

However, optimal health requires more than just exercise; nutrition also plays a critical role, influencing our energy levels, mood, and resilience.

Our dietary choices profoundly affect our body's response to stress, including cortisol levels, which can disrupt balance and contribute to health issues like weight gain and inflammation. To support our somatic therapy journey and mitigate the effects of cortisol, we must prioritize a balanced diet.

The DASH (Dietary Approaches to Stop Hypertension) diet, emphasizing nutrient-rich whole foods while limiting sodium and unhealthy fats, aligns well with somatic therapy principles. By nourishing our bodies with wholesome foods, we promote optimal health and vitality.

Additionally, the DASH diet's focus on reducing sodium intake can benefit stress-related issues like hypertension, complementing somatic therapy's stress-relieving effects.

In essence, integrating the dash diet with somatic therapy creates a synergistic approach to wellness, promoting balance, resilience, and vibrant well-being.

Scan the QR code here below to unlock a delightful bonus: free access to a selection of delicious recipes and a 30-day dash diet program. Enjoy the flavors of nourishing meals while embarking on your somatic therapy journey.

Conclusion

As we conclude our journey through somatic exercises, let's reflect on their profound impact on our well-being.

This book serves as a guide to understanding and practicing these exercises, which offer a holistic approach to integrating our mental, emotional, and physical selves.

They go beyond mere movements; they provide a pathway to deep self-awareness and transformation.

Throughout this book, we've explored exercises designed to alleviate pain, facilitate trauma recovery, release tension, reduce anxiety and stress, and improve posture. Each exercise builds upon the other, fostering harmony and balance within ourselves.

A central theme is the mind-body connection. Engaging in somatic exercises allows us to deepen our connection with our bodies and respond to them with compassion.

This awareness enhances our physical health and profoundly impacts our mental and emotional well-being.

Somatic exercises also address trauma, offering a compassionate means of releasing stored traumas, leading to a sense of liberation and renewal.

Embarking on this journey fosters qualities such as patience, mindfulness, and self-acceptance. Consistent practice is key to achieving lasting results, and integrating other aspects of well-being, such as nutrition, enhances effectiveness.

Somatic exercises serve as lifelong companions, adaptable to all stages of life. They offer a pathway to emotional balance, physical relief, and heightened self-awareness.

By engaging in them, we empower ourselves to take an active role in our own well-being.

In essence, somatic exercises offer opportunities for personal growth and restoration.

May your journey lead you to serenity, equilibrium, and profound inner connection. We hope the insights gained from this book support you in leading a more wholesome, peaceful, and balanced life.

Remember,
the path to wellness is continuous and each day brings you closer to a better version of yourself.

Thank you for choosing my book.

I really would like to hear your thoughts about your experience because your input is valuable and can inspire those who want to start this rewarding journey.
If you have a moment, please consider leaving a review.

Printed in Great Britain
by Amazon

44966387R00044